CONTENTS

Belly Diet Smoothies

Delicious Smoothie Recipes To Flatten Your Belly, Improve Your Gut & Burn Fat

LELA GIBSON

Introduction

I want to thank you and congratulate you for buying the book, *"Belly Diet Smoothies"*.

This book contains proven steps and strategies on how to flatten your belly, improve your gut and burn fat.

Let us face it, nowadays, many dubious and fraudulent manufacturers make products that use catch phrases or buzzwords such as "cleansing," "fat burning," or "detoxing". Unfortunately, there is no legitimate or scientific proof to show how such products work or if they work. Perhaps you have tried using "fat burning" juices and other drinks sourced from various fad diets only to end up losing your hard-earned money instead of body fat.

The good news is that weight loss through smoothies is not like other health and fitness gimmicks; it actually works. Besides being an effective way to lose excess body fat, smoothies eliminate the stress of cooking or needing to eat processed or packaged drinks that may contain unhealthy ingredients. Blending smoothies at home can be a cheap, easy, and quick way to supplement your diet with vegetables and fresh fruits, a nutritional element you could be missing.

If you are having doubts about integrating smoothies into your diet, or are unaware of which smoothie ingredients you should have, this book is for you. Here, you will learn the benefits of smoothies, how they encourage weight loss, and ingredients to incorporate into smoothies for weight loss.

Thanks again for buying this book, I hope you enjoy it!

Smoothies And Their Benefits

A healthy and nutritious smoothie comprises of a good balance of vitamins, proteins, healthy fats, and complex vegetables. That brings us to what makes a good weight loss smoothie. By default, a good weight-loss smoothie should be low in calories, and because it should be filling, it should:

Include fiber-rich foods

Choose foods such as chia seeds, flax meal, beans, pear, kiwi, avocado, kale, berries, bananas, and plant-based protein powders.

Have sufficient protein

While green smoothies are the best for weight loss, to help sustain energy production throughout the day, you need to feed your muscles. Avoid high-carbohydrate snacks but rather, add 10 grams of protein to each glass of smoothie. Ingredients such as nut butter, nuts, beans, soft tofu, protein powder, cottage cheese, and Greek yoghurt are perfect choices here.

Not have too much fruit

Thanks to their high fiber content and ample nutrients, fruits are healthier than processed carbohydrates. That said, some fruits are high in carbohydrates and calories; thus, the body breaks them down quickly triggering cravings for food 1-2 hours after eating. To combat hunger pangs, pair low-carbohydrate fruits with other ingredients such as soymilk, nut butter, or protein powder.

Not have sweeteners

The fact is that green smoothies could have an unpleasant taste; however, for obvious reasons, you should not add sweeteners. Ingredients such as maple syrup or honey can add at least an extra 60 calories to your smoothie. This addition makes weight loss harder. Avoid sweetened or flavored milk, yoghurt and fruits canned with syrup; instead, choose almond milk, soymilk, or plain yoghurt.

Before we look at some tasty smoothie recipes, you may probably be wondering why you should take smoothies especially belly diet smoothies in order to lose weight. This is why:

Belly Diet Smoothies promote satiety or fullness

Do you know that in order to lose weight, your body requires a higher supply of nutrients and minerals to provide required fuel to burn body fat? One of the best ways to help your metabolism get such nutrients is to eat ample fruits, dark-leafy green veggies, and a few complex carbohydrates that also promote satiety.

Healthy fruits and veggies help you increase fiber content intake. Fiber is important in absorbing fluids that contribute to "water weight" and takes up much space in the stomach to promote fullness. With increased satiety, you can effectively combat hunger and cravings for sweet and processed foods that hinder effective weight loss.

Furthermore, smoothies offer detox benefits. Consumption of fruits and veggies provides your body antioxidants, fiber, and phytonutrients that remove accumulated toxins from the body. Because of the effective detox effect, you will feel lighter and clear of mind without the need for fasting.

These Smoothies are low in calories

One unique feature of smoothies is that compared to most meals or juices, they are lower in calories, which is very important if you are trying to lose weight. As opposed to store-bought juices, homemade smoothies do not have added sugars. You probably already know that to trigger weight loss, you need to create a calorie deficit by consuming lesser calories than your metabolism can utilize. To do this, you do not have to eat less or starve yourself; instead, lower your intake of high carbohydrate foods that are also high in calories.

To burn fat, the body needs a specific minimum calorie intake to maintain current body weight and support metabolism and bodily functions in what we call *calorie maintenance level.* If you can supply your body with the exact calories it needs, chances are your body weight would never change. The body would utilize all the calories you eat and thus, it would have no extra amount to convert to body fat.

With a low calorie diet such as taking smoothies, you can effortlessly lose weight without having to work harder in the gym. In place of sugary and processed drinks such as non-diet sodas, go for satiating ingredients such as fresh fruits and non-starchy veggies that are low calorie.

Try incorporating low carbohydrate fruits such as avocados, apples, berries, pears, bananas, papayas, oranges, pineapples, among others. Also add dark leafy veggies such as spinach, cauliflower, Brussels sprouts, green beans, cabbage, lettuce, and asparagus among others.

Are great sources of probiotics

Smoothies also incorporate other healthy ingredients such as yoghurt, chocolate, and many others. Probiotics such as yoghurt have many health benefits such as improved gut health, weight loss, and improved immunity. Having a healthy gut is the key to living a disease free life since your intestinal health dictates how well you digest and utilize food.

Proper digestion facilitates absorption of nutrients as well as removal of toxins that contribute to weight gain. The gut also harbors more than 70 percent of immune cells, and thus helps protect you from infections. In other words, it serves as a host for friendly bacteria referred to as *Intestinal Flora.*

The beneficial bacteria help monitor your hormonal level, facilitate excretion of toxins, and synthesize substances that keep your intestines healthy. Since a majority of your immune cells lives in the gut, by interacting with these cells, the bacteria in the intestines help boost your immunity.

Incorporating yoghurt into your smoothies can help balance the gut bacteria by ensuring that beneficial bacteria outnumber the harmful bacteria. In such a case, you can effortlessly combat bacteria, viruses, and fight cancer promoting cells or other cancerous toxins.

Belly Diet Smoothie Tips

In order to enjoy your journey of losing belly fat by taking smoothies, you need to know a few things. Below are some tips that will be of great help as you get started with the smoothies:

Plan ahead

It's true that you want to burn fat and flatten your belly. This does not mean that you have all the time in the world to do so. Most people are just too busy to measure out ingredients and chop things up in the morning. This is not an excuse not to drink your smoothie at this time. You can prepare your smoothie ahead and freeze it in a muffin tin. Thus, when you wake up, you'll only need to pulse it for a few seconds and you're ready to go.

Also, it is good to note that you need to do your shopping beforehand to ensure you have all the ingredients you need. If you want to use fresh or organic ingredients, you must shop earlier. Make a list and determine which items can last for longer periods and which ones need to be frozen for later. Preparation will ensure you do not miss some ingredients when you want to make your smoothies.

Take care of your blades

Your blender can serve you well for a long time if you treat it well. If you intend to make smoothies for a long time, you'd do well to take care of your blades. When making smoothies, you can start by adding liquid, followed by soft fruits, then vegetables and finely ice. The liquid will lubricate the blades and this will enable them to have an easier time cutting through harder ingredients. If you protect your blades, you'll extend the lifespan of the blender, which will ensure the blender serves you for a longer time.

Put any surplus to good use

Don't be so quick to discard any surplus when you make smoothies. There are times you'll find a little bit of the smoothie remaining and since you wouldn't want to consume more than you should, you may be at a loss as to what to do. Well, you can put any remaining smoothies to good use by making popsicles out of them. You can place them in a popsicle mold or an ice tray or even paper cups. Add a toothpick to each mold and enjoy the popsicles when you want something to snack on instead of eating unhealthy snacks.

Use blending to your advantage when cleaning

Let's just say that cleaning your blender after you've made certain smoothies is no fun at all. You need to ensure you get all the little bits stuck at the bottom, which can be quite hard. However, there is another way to simplify your work. You can simply blend some water and dish washing soap. Once done, rinse the blender thoroughly and allow it to dry.

Keep an eye on the calories

One thing you'll discover as you try out various belly diet smoothies is that most of them are quite tasty. You may start making smoothies with the intention of flattening your belly only to end up putting on weight due to overindulging. Always keep in mind that fruits and vegetables contain calories. Actually, fruits are quite high in calories; therefore, it is advisable to balance the fruits and vegetables in your smoothie to ensure that the smoothie is not too high in calories, which can only lead to weight gain.

Freeze bananas

Bananas often make an appearance in quite a number of smoothie recipes. It is for this reason you need to have a bunch of them on hand in case you need them. Unfortunately, bananas to tend to go bad quickly. Thus, unless you intend to use them immediately, it would be best to freeze them. Frozen bananas add that extra kick to recipes.

In order to freeze bananas, first peel them and then cut them into smaller slices. Once you're done, quickly place them in zip lock bags and freeze them. This way, it would only be a matter of adding them to whatever ingredients you are blending whenever you need them.

Apart from freezing bananas, you can also freeze vegetables such as fresh kale and spinach. These vegetables are great especially when it comes to making green smoothies. Some people find it easier to freeze such vegetables in ice trays rather than zip lock bags. However, whichever way you freeze them, remember to do so quickly as you won't want them to spoil once you slice them.

Mix it up

Switch up the recipes so that you don't have to keep drinking the same thing over and over again unless you really like it. Making smoothies is an adventure; therefore, you should try out new stuff and discover new fruits and vegetables that you would otherwise never have tried. As they say, you shouldn't knock it before you try it.

If you want to try out making smoothies without a recipe, you can do so. But you should be cautious when it comes to adding liquids. Start by adding only a little liquid. This way, you can always add more if the smoothie is not to your desired consistency. If you start by adding a lot of liquid, you may have a hard time getting the desired consistency.

Enjoy the experience

Losing fat does not have to be boring. You can put some fun into your smoothie making experience. Why not put on some music and dance around as you get your smoothies ready? You can also have fun sharing the experience with others. Kids especially are more likely to drink smoothies if they helped in their preparation. It can also be a great teaching opportunity as you get to discuss topics to do with fruits and vegetables.

All in all, experiment and have fun while trying out various belly diet smoothie recipes.

The following chapter will provide numerous recipes that you can try out as you focus on losing belly fat.

Smoothie Recipes

Green Smoothie

Ingredients

1 tablespoon of flax seed oil

1 serving of green super-food powder

1 serving of protein powder

½ cup of frozen berries

1 banana

1 cup of kale, with stems removed

1 cup of baby spinach

2 cups of water

Some honey or stevia to sweeten, optional

Directions

Place a serving of green super-food powder, frozen berries, a banana, a cup of kale and baby spinach, water, and flax seed oil into your blender.

Blend the mixture until creamy.

You can add a little honey or stevia to sweeten the smoothie if you like. Serve and enjoy.

Aloe Vera Smoothie

Ingredients

1-2 aloe vera leaves, filleted

1 handful of fresh basil

½ cup of mango slices, fresh or frozen

½ cup of raspberries, fresh or frozen

2 cups of coconut milk or water

Directions

Place the basil, mango slices, raspberries, Aloe Vera, and coconut milk in a blender.

Process the mixture for minute or so until you achieve the desired thickness.

For extra sweetness, consider adding stevia or honey.

Cantaloupe Smoothie

Ingredients

6 ice cubes

1 cup of strawberries, frozen

2 cups of cantaloupe slices, chopped

10 large romaine lettuce leaves

Directions

Place the frozen strawberries, cantaloupe slices, romaine lettuce leaves, and ice cubes in a blender

Process until ready and serve.

Oatmeal Smoothie

Ingredients

½ cup of Greek yogurt, your favorite variety

2 tablespoons of flaxseed meal or flax seeds, ground

1 cup of milk

½ cup of oats, raw or unprepared

1 cup of ice

1 cup of blueberries

Directions

Layer ground flaxseeds and Greek yogurt, a cup of milk, unprepared oats, and blueberries in the blender.

To control the thickness of your smoothie, add more ice for thicker consistency or less for a thinner drink.

Coffee Replacement Smoothie

Ingredients

¼ teaspoon of vanilla powder

1 tablespoon of cacao powder

1 tablespoon of coconut oil

3 tablespoons of cashews

1 cup of almond milk

A little sea salt

Sweetener; honey or stevia, optional

Directions

Process the ingredients in a blender until smooth.

You can add a little sea salt and honey to improve taste.

Tropical Smoothie

Ingredients

¾ cup of fresh pineapple cubes

1 cup of spinach

2 tablespoons of coconut, shredded

4 or 5 ice cubes

¾ cup of coconut milk

6 ounces of Greek yogurt

Directions

Combine fresh pineapple cubes, spinach, shredded coconut, ice cubes and coconut milk along with the Greek yogurt in a blender.

Process the mixture until smooth.

Basic Green Smoothie

Ingredients

1 banana

1 bunch of baby spinach

1 cup of water

Directions

In a blender, add a bunch of baby spinach, a banana, a cup of water, and then process the mixture for a few seconds, serve and enjoy.

Apple Smoothie

Ingredients

1 red apple, cored and sliced into pieces

1 cup mixed berries

1 bunch baby spinach

Directions

Process all the ingredients in a blender until smooth. Serve and enjoy.

Apple Protein Smoothie

Ingredients

4 or 5 ice cubes

Pinch of cinnamon

Pinch of nutmeg

1 ounce of vanilla protein powder

12 ounces of almond milk

1 apple

Directions

In a blender or food processor, combine vanilla protein powder, cinnamon, nutmeg, almond milk, and a few ice cubes.

Process the mixture until smooth.

Almond Smoothie

Ingredients

½ cup of non-fat yogurt or almond milk

2 teaspoons of flaxseed

1 tablespoon of almond butter

1 banana, sliced and frozen

½ teaspoon of almond or vanilla extract

Directions

In a blender, add almond milk or low-fat yogurt, flaxseed, almond butter, frozen banana and some vanilla or almond extract.

Process the mixture until smooth and creamy. Serve and enjoy.

Berry Smoothie

Ingredients

¼ cup of Greek yogurt

½ cup of milk

3 or 4 ice cubes

1 cup mixed berries

Directions

Place the above ingredients in a blender starting with the berries then the yogurt, ice cubes, milk, and honey. Process the mixture until smooth.

Super-food Smoothie

Ingredients

1 serving of green super-food powder

1 serving of chocolate protein powder

1 tablespoon of cacao powder

1 tablespoon of Maca powder

½ avocado, peeled and sliced

1 cup of kefir

1 cup of milk

Directions

Place the ingredients in a blender and process for some time until smooth and then serve.

Spinach Raspberry Shake

Ingredients

¼ cup of oatmeal

2 scoops of vanilla protein powder

2 teaspoons of flaxseed oil

Handful of spinach, fresh

8 baby carrots

1 cup Greek yogurt

1 cup of frozen raspberries

12 ice cubes

Directions

Place the ice cubs, oatmeal, vanilla protein powder, flaxseed oil, fresh spinach, baby carrots, yogurt and frozen raspberries in a blender.

Blend this mixture until smooth.

Fruity Smoothie

Ingredients

½ cup of yogurt

¼ cup of blueberries, frozen

1 cup of peach slices, frozen

1 tablespoon of vanilla soy protein (if desired)

Directions

Place non-fat or fat-free yogurt, frozen blueberries, frozen peaches and some water into a blender and then process until smooth.

Add in a tablespoon of vanilla soy protein if you like. Finally, pour into a glass and enjoy.

Chocolate Strawberry Smoothie

Ingredients

½ teaspoon of Maca Powder

2 teaspoons of hemp seeds

1 tablespoon of chia seeds

2 tablespoon of cacao powder

1½ cups of almond milk

1 cup of strawberries, fresh or frozen

Directions

In a high-speed blender, combine all the above ingredients and then process at high speed until smooth.

Pour in a tall glass and enjoy.

Garnish with frozen cocoa nibs, hemp seeds, and frozen strawberries to add a different crunch.

Pomegranate Strawberry Smoothie

Ingredients

1 pomegranate

1 cup of pomegranate juice, unsweetened

1 ounce of whey protein powder

1½ cups of frozen berries strawberries

A banana, optional

Directions

Combine the pomegranate, unsweetened pomegranate juice, protein powder, berries and banana if you like.

Process the mixture until smooth and creamy.

The banana is great in helping to counter the strong taste of pomegranate.

Strawberry Smoothie

Ingredients

2 teaspoons of flaxseed oil, cold-pressed organic variety

1 cup of frozen strawberries, unsweetened

1 cup of milk

Directions

In a blender, combine frozen and unsweetened berries with a cup of skim milk.

After blending, pour the mixture in a glass and then add cold-pressed organic flaxseed oil, while stirring.

Enjoy your fat-burning drink.

Chocolate Fruit Smoothie

Ingredients

1 cup of water

1 tablespoon flaxseed

1 teaspoon of cocoa, unsweetened

½ cup of blueberries, frozen

4 or 5 ice cubes

1000 mg chitosan

A scoop of Whey protein

Directions

Combine the milled flaxseeds, unsweetened cocoa, frozen berries, chitosan, whey protein, and water in a blender.

Blend for a minute or so until smooth and creamy.

Chocolate (cocoa) is effective at burning fat or losing weight.

Pineapple Smoothie

Ingredients

1 tablespoon of flaxseed oil, cold-pressed and organic

4 ounce of pineapple tidbits in juice, canned

Handful of ice

1 cup of skim milk

1 handful baby spinach

Directions

Combine the spinach, skim milk, canned pineapple, and a few ice cubes in a blender and then blend for a minute or so.

When ready, transfer the smoothie to a glass and then add a tablespoon of cold-pressed and organic flaxseed oil.

Banana Cocoa Smoothie

Ingredients

1 tablespoon of honey

2 tablespoons of cocoa powder, unsweetened

½ cup of soymilk

½ cup of silken tofu

1 banana

Directions

Peel and slice a medium-sized banana and put it in a freezer or refrigerator until firm.

Blend the tofu, cocoa, honey, soymilk, and then add in the frozen banana slices. Continue blending until smooth.

Blueberry and Green Tea Smoothie

Ingredients

3 ice cubes

12 ounces of vanilla yogurt, fat free

2 cups of blueberries

2 tablespoons of almonds

2 tablespoons of flax seeds, ground

2 green tea bags

¾ cup of water to brew the tea.

Directions

Start by brewing the two green tea bags using a ¾ cupful of water and allow the mixture to cool.

Transfer the green tea to a blender and then add in vanilla yogurt, blueberries, ground flaxseeds, almonds, and ice cubes. Blend for a few seconds to achieve your desired thickness.

Mixed Berry Smoothie

Ingredients

2 cups of filtered water

1 teaspoon of organic stevia powder

Organic baby spinach, few handfuls

½ cup of organic Greek yogurt, non-fat

2 cups of mixed berries, fresh

Directions

Place some filtered water in a blender and then add in fat free Greek yogurt.

Add the other ingredients, blend the mixture to the desired thickness and enjoy.

Avocado Raspberry Smoothie

Ingredients

½ cup of raspberries, frozen

¾ cup of raspberry juice

1 peeled and pitted avocado

1 cup spinach

Directions

In a blender, combine the frozen raspberries, raspberry juice, peeled avocado and spinach.

Blend for a few seconds until smooth. Pour into a glass and enjoy.

Apple Pecan Smoothie

Ingredients

1 tablespoon of vanilla protein powder

3 to 4 ice cubes

1 cup of coconut milk, unsweetened

¼ cup pecans, unsalted

Dash of nutmeg

Dash of cinnamon

1 tablespoon of coconut butter

An apple, with the skin

Stevia liquid or another sweetener, few drops to taste

Directions

Add vanilla protein powder, ice cubes, unsweetened coconut milk, pecans, coconut butter, and apple.

Sprinkle some little cinnamon, nutmeg, and a sweetener such as stevia liquid if you like.

Blend the mixture until smooth and then pour into a glass to serve.

Lime Smoothie

Ingredients

8-10 ice cubes

½ cup of raspberries

1 cup of lime sherbet, low-fat

2/3 cup of skim milk

½ cup of lime, sliced

Directions

Put raspberries, low-fat lime sherbet, skim milk, lime, and ice cubes into a blender and then process to the desired thickness.

Pour your smoothie into a glass and enjoy this healthy and delicious drink.

Mixed Up Smoothie

Ingredients

6 ice cubes

1 handful baby spinach

1 orange, peeled

¼ cup of banana slices

¼ cup of apple slices

Directions

Place ice cubes, honey, banana slices, peeled orange, spinach and apple slices in your blender.

Process until smooth and enjoy.

Chocolate Almond Smoothie

Ingredients

1 serving of chocolate protein powder

2 tablespoons hemp seeds, flax or chia

2 tablespoons of almond butter

1 cup of cubed apple

2 cups of milk

Directions

Place the ingredients in your blender and process until you get your desired consistency.

Blueberry Milkshake

Ingredients

A dash of cinnamon

2 tablespoons of Maca powder

1 pinch sea salt

¼ teaspoon of vanilla powder

1 cup of blueberries, fresh or frozen

2 cups of milk

Directions

Add the vanilla powder, blueberries, sea salt, maca and a dash of cinnamon into your blender.

Process the ingredients until smooth.

Tomato Smoothie

Ingredients

8-10 ice cubes

½-1 teaspoon of hot sauce

¼ cup of celery, chopped

½ cup of carrots, chopped

¼ cup of apple juice

½ cup of tomato juice

2 cups of tomatoes, chopped

Directions

In a blender, put hot sauce, ice cubes, chopped celery, carrots, tomatoes, and orange juice.

Process until smooth and enjoy.

Chocolate Avocado Smoothie

Ingredients

1 serving of chocolate protein powder

2 tablespoons of cacao nibs or cacao powder

½ avocado, peeled and sliced

2 cups of milk

A few mint leaves, e.g. mint chocolate chip ice cream

A little honey or stevia to sweeten (optional)

Directions

Place all the ingredients in your blender and process for a few seconds until smooth.

Maca Smoothie

Ingredients

A dash of sea salt

1 banana

1 tablespoon of bee pollen

2 tablespoons of Maca powder

1½ cups of water

Directions

Add Maca powder, bee pollen, a banana, sea salt, and one and a half cups of water into your blender

Blend until smooth. Once done, pour into a glass and enjoy your smoothie.

Blueberry Smoothie

Ingredients

1 tablespoon of cold-pressed organic flaxseed oil

1 cup of frozen blueberries, unsweetened

1 cup of skim milk

Directions

In a blender, mix the blueberries and milk and puree for a minute.

Pour into a glass and stir in the flaxseed oil.

Banana and Peanut Butter Smoothie

Ingredients

4 ice cubes

¼ very ripe banana

2 tablespoons of creamy natural peanut butter, unsalted

½ cup of fat-free plain yogurt

½ cup of fat-free milk

Directions

Mix all the ingredients in a blender and process until smooth.

Pour the smoothie into a glass and enjoy your drink.

Chocolate Milkshake

Ingredients

3 ice cubes

1 cup of vanilla soymilk

1 tablespoon of flax meal

2 cups of spinach

¼ cup of fresh raspberries

½ frozen banana

1/8 cup of cocoa powder

½ package of silken tofu

Directions

Combine all the ingredients in a blender and process until smooth.

Pour in a glass and enjoy.

Carrot Smoothie

Ingredients

3 ice cubes

Dash of ground cloves

Dash of ground nutmeg

½ teaspoon of cinnamon

1/8 cup of golden raisins

½ scoop of vanilla protein powder

1 cup of unsweetened soymilk

2 cups of spinach

½ frozen banana

2 medium carrots, peeled and chopped

Directions

Combine everything in a blender then process until smooth.

Serve

Chia Berry Smoothie

Ingredients

½ tablespoon of chia seeds

½ cup of water

½ cup of pomegranate juice, unsweetened

1 cup of frozen mixed berries

Directions

Mix all the ingredients in a blender, process until smooth.

Pour the smoothie into a glass and garnish with some chia seeds.

Fiber and Protein-Rich Smoothie

Ingredients

¼ teaspoon of cinnamon

½ cup of nonfat milk

¾ cup of nonfat Greek yogurt

1 banana

1 red apple

5 raw almonds

Directions

Add all ingredients in a blender then puree for 30 seconds on high speed until smooth.

Note: You may have to chop the almonds and apples beforehand.

Papaya Smoothie

Ingredients

½ cup of fresh papaya

4 ice cubes

2 cups of spinach

1 cup of chilled coconut water

¼ cucumber (with skin)

1 frozen banana

½ cup of pineapple, fresh

Directions

Add all ingredients in a blender and process until smooth.

Serve and enjoy.

Tasty Spinach Smoothie

Ingredients

1 or 2 tablespoons of fresh lime juice

2 tablespoons of chopped avocado

6 ounces of fat-free plain Greek yogurt

15 green or red grapes

1 ripe pear, peeled, cored, and chopped

2 cups of spinach leaves, packed

Directions

Mix all the ingredients in a food processor or blender.

Puree until smooth or preferred consistency.

Flat-Belly Smoothie

Ingredients

¾ cup of water

1 cup of kale

½ cup of pineapple, frozen

½ cup of frozen blueberries

1 tablespoon of almond butter

3 ounces of vanilla nonfat Greek yogurt

Directions

Process all the ingredients in a blender, until smooth.

Pour the smoothie into a tall glass, garnish with blueberries and enjoy.

Banana Bread Smoothie

Ingredients

2 tablespoons of chopped walnuts

1 scoop of vanilla protein powder

½ medium banana (frozen or fresh)

½ cup of vanilla almond milk

½ cup of low-fat cottage cheese

½ teaspoon of nutmeg

1 teaspoon of cinnamon

½ teaspoon of vanilla extract

Directions

Add the ingredients to a blender, puree until smooth, and serve.

Vanilla Milkshake Smoothie

Ingredients

½ tablespoon of peanut butter

1 frozen banana

1 cup of vanilla soymilk

½ cup of soft tofu

Directions

Place the ingredients in a food processor or blender, puree until smooth and serve immediately.

Strawberry Yogurt Smoothie

Ingredients

3 ice cubes

12 raw almonds

1 cup of unsweetened soymilk

3 ounces of soy yogurt

½ cup of blueberries

½ banana

4 large strawberries

Directions

Add the ingredients to a food processor or blender and puree.

Once done, pour the creamy smoothie into a glass and enjoy.

Metabolism-Boosting Smoothie

Ingredients

¼ teaspoon of cinnamon

1 teaspoon of flax meal

¾ cup of iced green tea

¼ cup of cannellini or garbanzo beans

1 cup of frozen strawberries

¼ cup of broccoli florets with stems cut off

8 almonds

6 ounces of vanilla nonfat Greek yogurt

Directions

Mix all the ingredients in a blender and process until smooth.

Serve topped with a dash of cinnamon.

Skinny Green Smoothie

Ingredients

½ cup of plain fat-free Greek yogurt

¾ cup of vanilla almond milk, unsweetened

1 tablespoon of Peanut Butter

2 cups of baby spinach

1 small ripe banana, peeled and frozen

Directions

Combine fat-free yoghurt, almond milk, peanut butter, baby spinach, and frozen bananas in a blender.

Add in ice and then process until smooth.

For a variation, you can add in blueberries, protein powder, and flax seeds.

Cucumber Apple Smoothie

Ingredients

10 ice cubes

¼ cup of fresh mint, chopped

¼ cup of cold water

1/3 cup of 100% apple juice undiluted, unsweetened, and frozen

1 cup of chopped cucumber, seeded and peeled

Directions

Combine the ice cubes, cold water, apple juice concentrate, and a chopped cucumber in a blender and process until smooth..

When ready, pour the smoothie into your serving glass immediately and enjoy.

Green Smoothie

Ingredients

Juice from ½ lemon

2 cups of spinach, tightly packed

1 apple, cored

1 frozen banana, optional

1 cup of strawberries, frozen

1 cup of water

½ cup of chopped cucumber

Ice, optional

Directions

In a blender, combine 2 cups of freshly packed spinach with an apple, juice from half lemon, frozen strawberries, and a cup of water.

If you like, incorporate a frozen banana or additional ice. Process the ingredients until ready.

To lower the sugar or level of calories, omit one fruit serving and then add in some stevia/xylitol. You can add in a tablespoon of milled flaxseeds or chia seeds to get some healthy fats.

Breakfast Shake

Ingredients

¼ teaspoon of pure vanilla extract

Chai tea bag

½ teaspoon of cinnamon

½ teaspoon of ginger, powdered

1 cup of milk of choice

1 banana

Sweetener, optional

Directions

Start by brewing the tea using a chai tea bag and then cool the drink before blending.

Add the other ingredients into a blender: vanilla extract, cinnamon, ginger, ripe and frozen banana. Process until smooth, and then serve.

Berry & Yogurt Smoothie

Ingredients

1 teaspoon of agave nectar or honey

1 tablespoon of flax meal

¼ cup of skim milk

¼ cup of Greek yogurt, non-fat

½ banana

1 cup of berries of your choice

1½ cups of boiling water

1 green (or herbal) tea bag

Directions

Use the water to make 1 ½ cups of green tea. Ensure you allow the tea to steep for at least 10 minutes to increase concentration. When strongly concentrated, transfer the tea to an ice cube tray and then put in the freezer until solid.

Combine flax meal, agave nectar, Greek yoghurt, a banana, berries, and the green tea ice cubes (your frozen tea) and blend until smooth.

When ready, pour into your cup and enjoy.

Lemon Detox smoothie

Ingredients

Juice from 1 large orange

2 medium bananas (peeled)

½ medium lemon, (peeled and deseeded)

1-2 cups of chopped dandelion greens

½ medium lime, peeled and deseeded

Directions

Start by adding the liquid into your blender, followed by the soft fruit. The greens should go last.

Blend until creamy, or for about 30 seconds.

Raspberry Chia Smoothie

Ingredients

2 handfuls of ice or to your liking

Pinch of nutmeg

½ teaspoon of cinnamon

½ cup of water

1 scoop of protein powder

1 tablespoon of chia seeds

½ cup of plain Greek yogurt

½ cup of raspberries

½ banana

Directions

Place the ingredients apart from the ice in a high-speed blender and process until smooth. Add in 1-2 handfuls of ice and continue to pulse to smoothness.

Once done, pour into a glass and serve. Add more ice for a thicker smoothie or lesser in case you are using frozen berries or bananas.

Strawberry Protein Smoothie

Ingredients

1 cup of crushed ice

½ cup of fat free milk

1/3 cup of reduced fat cottage cheese

1-½ cups of fresh strawberries, quartered

Optional: 1 teaspoon of chia seeds

6 to 8 drops of liquid stevia

Directions

Preheat your oven to 425 degrees F. On a baking sheet lined with parchment paper, pour the strawberries and roast in the oven for 12-15 minutes.

Once the berries begin to release their juices, remove from the oven, and set aside.

Pour the roasted strawberries and their juice in a blender along with the chia seeds, ice, milk and cottage cheese and process until smooth.

Pour into a glass and serve.

Berry Smoothie

Ingredients

2 teaspoons of fresh lemon juice

1 teaspoon of flaxseed, ground

2 teaspoons of fresh ginger, finely grated

1½ tablespoons of honey

¼ cup of frozen pitted cherries or raspberries, unsweetened

¾ cup of chilled almond or rice milk, unsweetened

1 cup of frozen raspberries, unsweetened

Directions

Add the above ingredients into a blender along with lemon juice.

Blend until smooth and then serve and enjoy.

Watermelon Smoothie

Ingredients

2 cups of ice

¼ cup of fat-free milk

2 cups of watermelon, chopped

Directions

Blend watermelon and milk for 15 seconds until smooth.

Add in the ice and puree for an additional 20 seconds. If desired, add more ice and blend for 10 seconds to thicken the smoothie.

Pumpkin Latte

Ingredients

¼ teaspoon of nutmeg

¼ cup of espresso

1 cup of vanilla coconut milk

½ teaspoon of cinnamon

2 tablespoons of honey

1 tablespoon of flax seed

2 tablespoons of roasted pumpkin seeds

1 cup of roasted or baked pumpkin

Whipped Cream if desired

Directions

Into a high-powered blender such as a NutriBullet, mix the honey, cinnamon, flaxseed, pumpkin seeds, pumpkin, and process until smooth.

Pour the mixture into heat-safe cups and microwave on high heat for 45-90 seconds.

Stir in the espresso and pour into the mugs before you top each of them with a tablespoon of coconut milk alongside a little amount of nutmeg.

If desired, consider garnishing with whipped cream.

Spinach Protein Smoothie

Ingredients

¼ cup frozen pineapple

¼ cup frozen mango chunks

1 handful of spinach, washed

1 scoop vanilla protein powder

1 tablespoon chia seeds

1 tablespoon flax meal

½ frozen banana

Directions

Combine the ingredients in a blender and process until smooth.

Breakfast Smoothie

Ingredients

4 oz. Vanilla Greek yogurt

1 orange, peeled and segmented

1 frozen banana

1 cup frozen mixed berries

Directions

Combine all ingredients in a blender and process until smooth.

Almond Butter Smoothie

Ingredients

1 tablespoon unsweetened almond butter

1 ripe banana, peeled and frozen

1 tablespoon chia seeds

¾ cup unsweetened almond milk

Directions

Mix the ingredients in a blender and process until you get your desired consistency. Pour the smoothie into a glass and enjoy.

Grape Smoothie

Ingredients

½ cup frozen red grapes

1 banana, peeled and frozen

1/8 teaspoon ground cinnamon

¼ cup orange juice

1 cup unsweetened almond milk

3 ice cubes

½ cup blueberries

Directions

Add all the ingredients into a blender and process until smooth.

Oat Berry Smoothie

Ingredients

½ cup old fashioned rolled oats

¼ cup ice

½ cup vanilla yogurt

3 tablespoons honey

½ cup frozen berries

1 cup milk

Directions

Put all the ingredients into your blender and process until smooth. Taste and add more honey to sweeten it or you can add more milk to make it thicker.

Peach and Oat Smoothie

Ingredients

½ cup water

½ cup oats

1 ripe banana, peeled and frozen

5.3 oz. Greek yogurt

1 cup almond milk

1 ½ cups peeled and diced peaches

Directions

Put all the ingredients in a blender and process until smooth and creamy.

I need your help...

Thank you again for buying this book! I hope this book was able to help you to get an idea of how to flatten your belly, improve your gut and burn fat.

The next step is to take action.

Finally, if you enjoyed this book, then I'd like to ask you for a favor, would you be kind enough to leave a review for this book on Amazon? It'd be greatly appreciated!

Please a review for this book on Amazon!

I want to reach as many people as I can with this book, and more reviews will help me accomplish that!

If you have any questions or problems, please contact us: hello@freedomdestination.com

Thank you and good luck!

Preview Of 'Anti-Inflammatory Diet Guide'

Effects Of Inflammation

Inflammation is the biological response your body goes into when dealing with harmful stimuli such as irritants, pathogens or even damaged cells. It is a self-protection mechanism that allows your body to begin the healing process. The 'hotness' or 'inflammation' you feel after you cut yourself or injure yourself is the result of your body working hard to heal itself. But what happens when your body experiences 'too much' inflammation?

A little inflammation is not a bad thing. In fact, when it happens, you should rejoice in knowing that your body is working tirelessly to correct the situation. However, like most good things, inflammation can get out of hand. When this happens, you may experience various health complications such as:

Weight Gain

Every day, thousands of people try to lose weight to no avail. They complain that they've tried out various diets but somehow none seem to be working. If they do find something that works, sooner than later, they are back to gaining the weight they thought they'd lost. This is because they neglect to look into inflammation as the cause for their weight gain. Inflammation contributes to weight gain in various ways. These include:

- If inflammation happens in the brain, it interferes with the functioning of the hypothalamus and this in turn increases your appetite and slows down your metabolism. When this happens, you will be eating a lot but burning up less energy, which leads to weight gain.

- Gut inflammation leads to leptin and insulin resistance. Leptin is the satiety hormone that tells your brain when you have had enough. When suffering from leptin resistance, you just eat and eat some more before leptin can communicate that you have had enough, which leads to weight gain. Another thing that gut inflammation does is to increase intestinal permeability. When this happens, more toxins will be able to permeate your bloodstream. Usually toxins are stored in fat cells to remove them from circulation. The more toxins you have, the more the fat cells expand to accommodate the more toxins leading to weight gain.

- Inflammation in the endocrine system suppresses adrenal and thyroid function. One of the main functions of the adrenal gland is to burn fat. Therefore, when you suppress the functioning of the adrenal gland, you are unable to burn fat, as you should leading to weight gain.

As you have read, inflammation is bad for you if you want to maintain the ideal weight.

Metabolic Syndrome

Metabolic syndrome refers to a group/cluster of lifestyle-related diseases including cardiovascular disease and obesity. They are clustered together because all of these diseases are linked to metabolic dysfunction. Markers of metabolic dysfunction include:

- Central obesity – this is excessive tummy fat

- Hyperinsulinaemia – this refers to ongoing high levels of insulin

- Insulin resistance –your body loses sensitivity to insulin (you need more insulin to manage your blood sugar levels)

But the question is how these three factors are connected. Well, when on a diet high in carbohydrates, your blood sugar levels increase leading to high insulin levels to help blood cells absorb the glucose and thus manage your blood sugar levels. When you have high insulin levels, the production of cytokines (which are pro-inflammatory) increases and in turn this causes inflammation especially in predisposed persons. Once inflammation increases, it brings with it an increase in the production of free radicals. Free radicals affect cellular functions and one of those functions just happens to be insulin sensitivity. This is why chronic low-grade inflammation is linked to all three markers; that is, raised insulin levels, obesity and decreased insulin sensitivity.

Chronic Fatigue

Many people suffering from chronic fatigue have been told that the disease 'is all in their minds'. Fortunately, in recent years more researchers have began looking into the association of chronic fatigue and inflammation. This is mainly because the two possess many similar symptoms including muscular pain and tenderness, sore throat, joint pain, swollen lymph nodes and sore throat.

As you know, inflammation is the way your body reacts to foreign particles. When you have symptoms of inflammation, it is safe to say that your body is fighting something even if that something is not yet known. This is why researchers link an overactive immune system to chronic fatigue.

Another thing that associates chronic fatigue with inflammation is the lack of cortisol in patients suffering from chronic fatigue. Cortisol is known to suppress inflammation. Thus, if your body has a cortisol deficiency, it will not be able to suppress inflammation and this will worsen symptoms of chronic fatigue. A dietary change often helps people suffering from chronic fatigue.

Some types of arthritis

When you hear the name arthritis, you automatically associate it with pain. Well, it is no coincidence since arthritis refers to inflammation in joints. When your joints experience inflammation, you will feel pain. The types of arthritis that have been linked to inflammation include:

- Gouty arthritis

- Rheumatoid arthritis

- Psoriatic arthritis

- Systematic lupus erythematosus

When you suffer from these types of arthritis, you may experience inflammation symptoms such as redness, joint stiffness, swelling of the joints, pain in the joints and loss of joint function.

It is important to note that inflammation does not have to be painful for it to be present. This is because many organs in your body just don't have enough pain-sensitive areas for you to feel that inflammatory sensation. This means that you can suffer from chronic inflammation over time without knowing, only for you to experience the effects of inflammation.

It is also important to note that various things can cause inflammation including:

- Processed foods high in sugar and unhealthy fats

- Omega-6 fats (and not enough Omega-3 fatty acids)

- Sleep deprivation

- Chronic stress

- Smoking

- Pollution

- Environmental chemicals

- Lack of exercise

Thus, chances are, if you experience any of the above things, you may be suffering from inflammation whether or not you experience pain.

The first thing you should do once you notice that you suffer from inflammation is not to reach for drugs because drugs just address the symptoms and not the root cause but rather to make some lifestyle changes. This is because most of the causes of inflammation can be addressed by making lifestyle changes like exercising more, reducing exposure to pollutants, not smoking and dietary changes.

In this book, we will focus on addressing inflammation by adopting an anti-inflammatory diet. Let us learn more about anti-inflammatory diet in the next chapter.

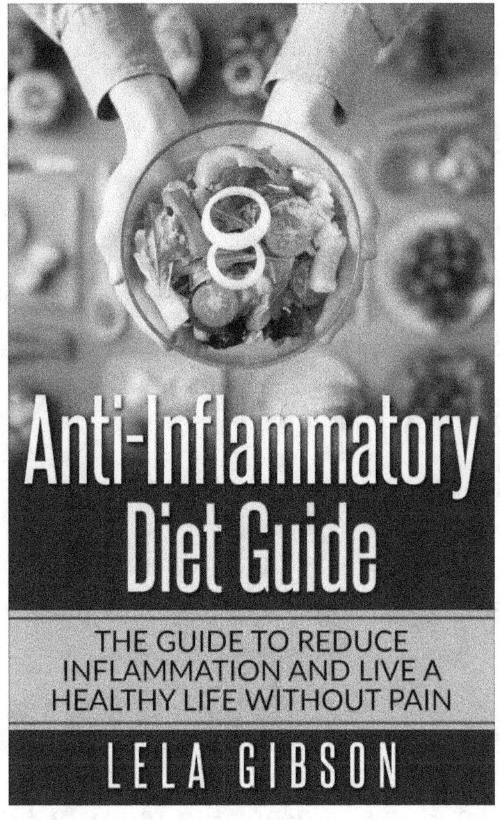

Check out the rest of Anti-Inflammatory Diet Guide on Amazon, go to: http://amzn.to/2qKTSPa

Check Out My Other Books

Below you'll find some of my other popular books that are popular on Amazon and Kindle as well.

Alternatively, you can visit my author page on Amazon to see other work done by me.

Belly Diet: The Zero Belly Diet Step-By-Step Guide Which Help You To Loose Your Belly And Enjoy Your Flat Belly

Anti-Inflammatory Diet Guide: The Guide To Reduce Inflammation And Live A Healthy Life Without Pain

Negative Calorie Diet: Cookbook & Guide Which Will Help You To Burn Body Fat, Lose Weight And Live Healthy

Clean Eating: Cookbook And Guide To Restore Your Body's Natural Balance And Eat Healthy

Dash Diet: Cookbook For Weight Loss With Action Plan And Easy Recipes

Freedom: How To Make Money Online And Become Financially Free By Creating Passive Income

Weight Loss: 20 Easy And Fast Diet Tips For Losing Weight – An Easy-To-Follow Weight Loss Guide

Smart Fat: Cookbook With Fat Meals Which Help You To Lose Weight, Get Healthy And Improve Brain Function

www.ingramcontent.com/pod-product-compliance
Lightning Source LLC
Chambersburg PA
CBHW070029260726
48658CB00002B/554